Smoothie For Weight Loss
And Good Health

RYLAN DAVIS

Disclaimer

Kindly note that the content in this book is basically for educational purposes. The information offered here is said to be reliable and can be trusted. The author makes no implication or intends to offer any warranty of accuracy for particular individual cases.
Before beginning any diet or lifestyle habits, it is recommended that you contact a knowledgeable practitioner, such as your physician. This book's material should not be utilized in place of expert counsel or professional guidance.
The author, publisher, and distributor expressly disclaim all liability, loss, damage, or danger incurred by persons who rely on the information in this book, whether directly or indirectly.
All intellectual property rights are retained. This book's information should not be replicated in any way, mechanically, electronically, photocopying, or by any other methods accessible.

Table of Contents

RECIPES

Green Detox Delight

Intro: Begin your day with a burst of green energy! The Green Detox Delight is a refreshing and nutrient-packed smoothie that aids in detoxification and supports overall well-being.

Total Prep Time: 5 minutes

Ingredients:
- 1 cup spinach leaves
- 1/2 cucumber, peeled and sliced
- 1 green apple, cored and chopped
- 1/2 lemon, juiced
- 1 cup coconut water
- Ice cubes (optional)

Instructions:
1. Place all ingredients in a blender.
2. Blend until smooth.
3. Pour into a glass and enjoy immediately.

Nutritional Information:
Calories: 120 | Protein: 3g | Fat: 1g | Carbohydrates: 30g | Fiber: 6g

Berry Bliss Booster

Intro: Indulge in the sweet and vibrant flavors of mixed berries with the Berry Bliss Booster. Packed with antioxidants, this smoothie is a delightful treat that supports your immune system.

Total Prep Time: 7 minutes

Ingredients:
- 1/2 cup strawberries, hulled
- 1/2 cup blueberries
-
- 1/2 cup raspberries
- 1/2 cup blackberries
- 1 cup Greek yogurt
- 1 tablespoon honey
- Ice cubes (optional)

Instructions:
1. Combine all berries, Greek yogurt, and honey in a blender.
2. Blend until creamy and smooth.
3. Pour into a glass and savor the berry bliss.

Nutritional Information:
Calories: 180 | Protein: 8g | Fat: 2g | Carbohydrates: 35g | Fiber: 7g

Tropical Slimming Shake

Intro: Transport yourself to the tropics with this Tropical Slimming Shake. Packed with tropical fruits and metabolism-boosting ingredients, this smoothie is a delicious way to support your weight loss journey.

Total Prep Time: 8 minutes

Ingredients:

- 1 cup pineapple chunks
- 1/2 banana
- 1/2 mango, peeled and diced
- 1 tablespoon chia seeds
- 1 cup coconut water
- Ice cubes (optional)

Instructions:

1. Combine pineapple, banana, mango, chia seeds, and coconut water in a blender.
2. Blend until smooth and creamy.
3. Pour into a glass, kick back, and enjoy the tropical vibes.

Nutritional Information:

Calories: 220 | Protein: 4g | Fat: 3g | Carbohydrates: 45g | Fiber: 9g

Cucumber Mint Refresher

Intro: Refresh your senses with the Cucumber Mint Refresher. This hydrating and invigorating smoothie is perfect for a hot day, providing a cooling sensation with every sip.

Total Prep Time: 6 minutes

Ingredients:

- 1 cucumber, peeled and sliced
- 1/2 cup fresh mint leaves
- 1 green apple, cored and chopped
- 1 tablespoon lime juice

- 1 cup water
- Ice cubes (optional)

Instructions:
1. Place cucumber, mint leaves, apple, lime juice, and water in a blender.
2. Blend until well combined and smooth.
3. Pour into a glass, garnish with mint, and enjoy the refreshing taste.

Nutritional Information:
Calories: 85 | Protein: 1g | Fat: 0g | Carbohydrates: 22g | Fiber: 4g

Blueberry Kale Power Smoothie

Intro: Fuel your body with a nutritional powerhouse – the Blueberry Kale Power Smoothie. Packed with vitamins and antioxidants, this smoothie is a tasty way to boost your energy levels.

Total Prep Time: 7 minutes

Ingredients:
- 1/2 cup blueberries
- 1 cup kale, stems removed
- 1/2 banana
- 1 tablespoon almond butter
- 1 cup almond milk
- Ice cubes (optional)

***Instructions**:*
1. Combine blueberries, kale, banana, almond butter, and almond milk in a blender.
2. Blend until smooth and creamy.
3. Pour into a glass and relish the nutritious goodness.

***Nutritional Information**:*
Calories: 150 | Protein: 5g | Fat: 7g | Carbohydrates: 20g | Fiber: 6g

Avocado Spinach Elixir

Intro: Experience a velvety, green elixir with the Avocado Spinach Elixir. Packed with healthy fats and leafy greens, this smoothie is a delicious way to nourish your body.

***Total Prep Time**:* 6 minutes

***Ingredients**:*
- 1/2 avocado, peeled and pitted
- 1 cup spinach leaves
- 1/2 cup pineapple chunks
- 1 tablespoon flaxseeds
- 1 cup coconut water
- Ice cubes (optional)

***Instructions**:*
1. Combine avocado, spinach, pineapple, flaxseeds, and coconut water in a blender.
2. Blend until creamy and smooth.
3. Pour into a glass, and enjoy the creamy texture and rich flavor.

Calories: 200 | Protein: 4g | Fat: 10g | Carbohydrates: 25g | Fiber: 8g

Pineapple Ginger Zing

Intro: Wake up your taste buds with the Pineapple Ginger Zing. This invigorating smoothie combines the tropical sweetness of pineapple with the spicy kick of ginger, creating a zesty flavor explosion.

Total Prep Time: 5 minutes

Ingredients:
- 1 cup pineapple chunks
- 1 tablespoon fresh ginger, grated
- 1/2 banana
- 1 tablespoon honey
- 1 cup water
- Ice cubes (optional)

Instructions:
1. Combine pineapple, fresh ginger, banana, honey, and water in a blender.
2. Blend until smooth and zesty.
3. Pour into a glass, garnish with a pineapple slice, and enjoy the zingy goodness.

Nutritional Information:
Calories: 140 | Protein: 1g | Fat: 0.5g | Carbohydrates: 35g | Fiber: 4g

Citrus Burst Metabolism Boost

Intro*:* Give your metabolism a kick-start with the Citrus Burst Metabolism Boost. This tangy and refreshing smoothie combines citrus fruits with metabolism-boosting ingredients to rev up your energy levels.

Total Prep Time*:* 7 minutes

Ingredients*:*
- 1 orange, peeled and segmented
- 1/2 grapefruit, peeled and segmented
- 1/2 lemon, juiced
- 1 tablespoon chia seeds
- 1 cup coconut water
- Ice cubes (optional)

Instructions*:*
1. Combine orange segments, grapefruit segments, lemon juice, chia seeds, and coconut water in a blender.
2. Blend until the mixture is smooth and bursting with citrus flavors.
3. Pour into a glass and enjoy the refreshing boost.

Nutritional Information*:*
Calories: 160 | Protein: 4g | Fat: 3g | Carbohydrates: 30g | Fiber: 8g

Almond Joy Protein Smoothie

Intro*:* Satisfy your sweet cravings guilt-free with the Almond Joy Protein Smoothie. This delightful smoothie combines the flavors of almond, coconut, and chocolate for a tasty and protein-packed treat.

Total Prep Time*:* 6 minutes

Ingredients*:*
- 1/2 cup almonds, soaked
- 1/4 cup shredded coconut
- 1 tablespoon cacao powder
- 1 banana
- 1 cup almond milk
- Ice cubes (optional)

Instructions*:*
1. Combine soaked almonds, shredded coconut, cacao powder, banana, and almond milk in a blender.
2. Blend until smooth and creamy.
3. Pour into a glass and relish the satisfying taste of this Almond Joy-inspired smoothie.

Nutritional Information*:*
Calories: 250 | Protein: 8g | Fat: 15g | Carbohydrates: 28g | Fiber: 7g

Watermelon Basil Fat Burner

Intro*:* Stay refreshed and support your weight loss journey with the Watermelon Basil Fat Burner. This hydrating smoothie combines the sweetness of watermelon with the aromatic essence of basil for a delightful experience.

Total Prep Time: 5 minutes

Ingredients:
- 1 cup watermelon, diced
- 1/4 cup fresh basil leaves
- 1/2 lime, juiced
- 1 tablespoon chia seeds
- 1 cup water
- Ice cubes (optional)

Instructions:
1. Combine watermelon, fresh basil, lime juice, chia seeds, and water in a blender.
2. Blend until smooth and refreshing.
3. Pour into a glass, garnish with a basil leaf, and enjoy the hydrating and fat-burning benefits.

Nutritional Information:
Calories: 90 | Protein: 2g | Fat: 3g | Carbohydrates: 18g | Fiber: 4g

Mango Tango Fat Flush

Intro: Kickstart your metabolism with the Mango Tango Fat Flush. This tropical delight combines the sweetness of mango with fat-flushing ingredients, making it a flavorful companion on your weight loss journey.

Total Prep Time: 6 minutes

Ingredients:
- 1 cup mango chunks
- 1/2 cup pineapple chunks
- 1 tablespoon flaxseeds
- 1/2 teaspoon cayenne pepper
- 1 cup coconut water
- Ice cubes (optional)

Instructions:
1. Combine mango, pineapple, flaxseeds, cayenne pepper, and coconut water in a blender.
2. Blend until smooth and tangy.
3. Pour into a glass and savor the tropical fat-flushing goodness.

Nutritional Information:
Calories: 140 | Protein: 2g | Fat: 3g | Carbohydrates: 30g | Fiber: 6g

Peachy Green Protein Punch

Intro: Elevate your protein intake with the Peachy Green Protein Punch. This smoothie combines the sweetness of peaches with the nutritional powerhouse of greens and protein, making it an ideal post-workout refuel.

Total Prep Time: 8 minutes

Ingredients:
- 1 cup peaches, sliced

- 1 cup spinach leaves
- 1/2 cup Greek yogurt
- 1 tablespoon hemp seeds
- 1 cup almond milk
- Ice cubes (optional)

Instructions:
1. Combine peaches, spinach, Greek yogurt, hemp seeds, and almond milk in a blender.
2. Blend until smooth and protein-packed.
3. Pour into a glass and enjoy the Peachy Green Protein Punch.

Nutritional Information:
Calories: 200 | Protein: 10g | Fat: 5g | Carbohydrates: 30g | Fiber: 6g

Raspberry Chia Seed Slimmer

Intro: Slim down with the Raspberry Chia Seed Slimmer. Packed with fiber and antioxidants, this smoothie is a delicious way to support weight loss and maintain a healthy metabolism.

Total Prep Time: 7 minutes

Ingredients:
- 1/2 cup raspberries
- 1 tablespoon chia seeds
- 1/2 banana
- 1 tablespoon honey
- 1 cup almond milk
- Ice cubes (optional)

Instructions:
1. Combine raspberries, chia seeds, banana, honey, and almond milk in a blender.
2. Blend until smooth and slimming.
3. Pour into a glass, garnish with a few raspberries, and enjoy the Raspberry Chia Seed Slimmer.

Nutritional Information:
Calories: 160 | Protein: 3g | Fat: 4g | Carbohydrates: 28g | Fiber: 8g

Spinach Pineapple Paradise

Intro: Transport yourself to a tropical paradise with the Spinach Pineapple Paradise. This green smoothie combines the goodness of spinach with the sweetness of pineapple, creating a refreshing and nutrient-packed drink.

Total Prep Time: 5 minutes

Ingredients:
- 1 cup spinach leaves
- 1 cup pineapple chunks
- 1/2 lime, juiced
- 1 tablespoon chia seeds
- 1 cup coconut water
- Ice cubes (optional)

Instructions:
1. Combine spinach, pineapple, lime juice, chia seeds, and coconut water in a blender.
2. Blend until smooth and paradise-worthy.

3. Pour into a glass and enjoy the refreshing taste of the Spinach Pineapple Paradise.

Nutritional Information:
Calories: 120 | Protein: 3g | Fat: 2g | Carbohydrates: 25g | Fiber: 6g

Chocolate Banana Protein Bliss

Intro: Satisfy your chocolate cravings while fueling your body with the Chocolate Banana Protein Bliss. This smoothie is a delightful blend of chocolatey goodness, banana sweetness, and protein power.

Total Prep Time: 6 minutes

Ingredients:
- 1 banana
- 1 tablespoon cacao powder
- 1 scoop chocolate protein powder
- 1 tablespoon almond butter
- 1 cup almond milk
- Ice cubes (optional)

Instructions:
1. Combine banana, cacao powder, chocolate protein powder, almond butter, and almond milk in a blender.
2. Blend until smooth and blissfully chocolatey.
3. Pour into a glass and relish the Chocolate Banana Protein Bliss.

Nutritional Information:
Calories: 250 | Protein: 20g | Fat: 8g |
Carbohydrates: 30g | Fiber: 7g

Pomegranate Blueberry Antioxidant Blend

Intro: Boost your antioxidant intake with the Pomegranate Blueberry Antioxidant Blend. This vibrant smoothie is rich in antioxidants, promoting cellular health and supporting your overall well-being.

Total Prep Time: 7 minutes

Ingredients:
- 1/2 cup pomegranate seeds
- 1/2 cup blueberries
- 1/2 cup strawberries, hulled
- 1 tablespoon acai powder
- 1 cup coconut water
- Ice cubes (optional)

Instructions:
1. Combine pomegranate seeds, blueberries, strawberries, acai powder, and coconut water in a blender.
2. Blend until smooth and bursting with antioxidants.
3. Pour into a glass and enjoy the Pomegranate Blueberry Antioxidant Blend.

Nutritional Information:
Calories: 160 | Protein: 2g | Fat: 1g |
Carbohydrates: 38g | Fiber: 9g

Kiwi Kale Cleanse

Intro: Cleanse and rejuvenate with the Kiwi Kale Cleanse. This green powerhouse smoothie combines the tartness of kiwi with the detoxifying benefits of kale, creating a refreshing and cleansing drink.

Total Prep Time: 6 minutes

Ingredients:
- 2 kiwis, peeled and sliced
- 1 cup kale, stems removed
- 1/2 cucumber, peeled and sliced
- 1 tablespoon lemon juice
- 1 cup water
- Ice cubes (optional)

Instructions:
1. Combine kiwi, kale, cucumber, lemon juice, and water in a blender.
2. Blend until smooth and cleansing.
3. Pour into a glass, garnish with a kiwi slice, and enjoy the Kiwi Kale Cleanse.

Nutritional Information:
Calories: 100 | Protein: 3g | Fat: 1g |
Carbohydrates: 25g | Fiber: 7g

Acai Berry Energizer

Intro: Revitalize your energy levels with the Acai Berry Energizer. Packed with the goodness of acai berries and other energizing ingredients, this smoothie is the perfect pick-me-up for any time of day.

Total Prep Time: 7 minutes

Ingredients:
- 1/2 cup acai berries (frozen or puree)
- 1/2 cup strawberries, hulled
- 1/2 banana
- 1 tablespoon chia seeds
- 1 cup almond milk
- Ice cubes (optional)

Instructions:
1. Combine acai berries, strawberries, banana, chia seeds, and almond milk in a blender.
2. Blend until smooth and energizing.
3. Pour into a glass and enjoy the Acai Berry Energizer.

Nutritional Information:
Calories: 180 | Protein: 4g | Fat: 5g | Carbohydrates: 30g | Fiber: 8g

Detoxifying Beet Berry Blast

Intro*:* Detoxify your body with the vibrant Detoxifying Beet Berry Blast. This smoothie combines the earthiness of beets with the sweetness of berries for a nutrient-packed blast of flavor.

Total Prep Time*:* 8 minutes

Ingredients:
- 1/2 cup beets, peeled and diced
- 1/2 cup mixed berries (blueberries, raspberries, blackberries)
- 1/2 cup pineapple chunks
- 1 tablespoon flaxseeds
- 1 cup coconut water
- Ice cubes (optional)

Instructions:
1. Combine beets, mixed berries, pineapple, flaxseeds, and coconut water in a blender.
2. Blend until smooth and detoxifying.
3. Pour into a glass and enjoy the nutrient-packed Detoxifying Beet Berry Blast.

Nutritional Information:
Calories: 150 | Protein: 3g | Fat: 3g | Carbohydrates: 30g | Fiber: 7g

Orange Carrot Revitalizer

Intro: Revitalize your body with the Orange Carrot Revitalizer. This smoothie blends the zesty flavor of oranges with the goodness of carrots for a revitalizing and immune-boosting drink.

Total Prep Time: 6 minutes

Ingredients:
- 2 oranges, peeled and segmented
- 1/2 cup carrots, peeled and sliced
- 1/2 inch ginger, grated
- 1 tablespoon honey
- 1 cup water
- Ice cubes (optional)

Instructions:
1. Combine oranges, carrots, ginger, honey, and water in a blender.
2. Blend until smooth and revitalizing.
3. Pour into a glass, garnish with an orange slice, and enjoy the Orange Carrot Revitalizer.

Nutritional Information:
Calories: 120 | Protein: 2g | Fat: 1g | Carbohydrates: 28g | Fiber: 5g

Coconut Lime Cooler

Intro*:* Chill out with the refreshing Coconut Lime Cooler. This tropical-inspired smoothie combines the creaminess of coconut with the zesty kick of lime for a cooling and hydrating experience.

Total Prep Time*:* 5 minutes

Ingredients*:*
- 1/2 cup coconut milk
- 1/2 cup coconut water
- 1 lime, juiced
- 1 tablespoon shredded coconut
- 1 cup ice cubes

Instructions*:*
1. Combine coconut milk, coconut water, lime juice, shredded coconut, and ice cubes in a blender.
2. Blend until smooth and refreshing.
3. Pour into a glass, garnish with a lime wedge, and enjoy the Coconut Lime Cooler.

Nutritional Information*:*
Calories: 120 | Protein: 1g | Fat: 8g | Carbohydrates: 10g | Fiber: 2g

Strawberry Basil Beauty

Intro*:* Enhance your natural beauty from the inside out with the Strawberry Basil Beauty smoothie. This antioxidant-rich blend combines the sweetness of strawberries with the aromatic essence of basil for a delightful treat.

Total Prep Time*:* 6 minutes

Ingredients*:*
- 1 cup strawberries, hulled
- 1/2 cup basil leaves
- 1/2 cup Greek yogurt
- 1 tablespoon honey
- 1 cup water
- Ice cubes (optional)

Instructions*:*
1. Combine strawberries, basil leaves, Greek yogurt, honey, and water in a blender.
2. Blend until smooth and beauty-enhancing.
3. Pour into a glass, garnish with a basil leaf, and enjoy the Strawberry Basil Beauty.

Nutritional Information*:*
Calories: 140 | Protein: 5g | Fat: 2g | Carbohydrates: 25g | Fiber: 4g

Pineapple Turmeric Tonic

Intro: Boost your immune system with the Pineapple Turmeric Tonic. This anti-inflammatory smoothie combines the tropical sweetness of pineapple with the golden goodness of turmeric for a tonic that promotes overall well-being.

Total Prep Time: 7 minutes

Ingredients:
- 1 cup pineapple chunks
- 1/2 teaspoon turmeric powder
- 1/2 banana
- 1 tablespoon chia seeds
- 1 cup coconut water
- Ice cubes (optional)

Instructions:
1. Combine pineapple, turmeric powder, banana, chia seeds, and coconut water in a blender.
2. Blend until smooth and immune-boosting.
3. Pour into a glass and enjoy the Pineapple Turmeric Tonic.

Nutritional Information:
Calories: 160 | Protein: 3g | Fat: 3g | Carbohydrates: 30g | Fiber: 7g

Cherry Almond Protein Fuel

Intro: Power up your day with the Cherry Almond Protein Fuel smoothie. This protein-packed blend combines the tartness of cherries with the nutty goodness of almonds for a satisfying and energizing drink.

Total Prep Time: 6 minutes

Ingredients:
- 1/2 cup cherries, pitted
- 1/4 cup almonds
- 1 scoop vanilla protein powder
- 1/2 banana
- 1 cup almond milk
- Ice cubes (optional)

Instructions:
1. Combine cherries, almonds, vanilla protein powder, banana, and almond milk in a blender.
2. Blend until smooth and protein-fueled.
3. Pour into a glass and enjoy the Cherry Almond Protein Fuel.

Nutritional Information:
Calories: 230 | Protein: 20g | Fat: 10g | Carbohydrates: 25g | Fiber: 6g

Mango Mint Metabolic Booster

Intro: Give your metabolism a refreshing boost with the Mango Mint Metabolic Booster. This smoothie combines the tropical sweetness of mango with the invigorating essence of mint for a revitalizing experience.

Total Prep Time: 5 minutes

Ingredients:
- 1 cup mango chunks
- 1/4 cup fresh mint leaves
- 1/2 lime, juiced
- 1 tablespoon honey
- 1 cup water
- Ice cubes (optional)

Instructions:
1. Combine mango, fresh mint, lime juice, honey, and water in a blender.
2. Blend until smooth and metabolism-boosting.
3. Pour into a glass, garnish with a mint sprig, and enjoy the Mango Mint Metabolic Booster.

Nutritional Information:
Calories: 140 | Protein: 1g | Fat: 0.5g | Carbohydrates: 35g | Fiber: 4g

Papaya Passion Fat Melter

Intro: Melt away the excess with the Papaya Passion Fat Melter. This tropical smoothie combines the tropical sweetness of papaya with passion fruit for a delightful drink that supports your weight loss goals.

Total Prep Time: 6 minutes

Ingredients:
- 1 cup papaya, diced
- 1/2 cup passion fruit pulp
- 1/2 banana
- 1 tablespoon chia seeds
- 1 cup coconut water
- Ice cubes (optional)

Instructions:
1. Combine papaya, passion fruit pulp, banana, chia seeds, and coconut water in a blender.
2. Blend until smooth and fat-melting.
3. Pour into a glass and enjoy the Papaya Passion Fat Melter.

Nutritional Information:
Calories: 150 | Protein: 2g | Fat: 2g | Carbohydrates: 35g | Fiber: 7g

Blueberry Avocado Immunity Infusion

Intro: Boost your immune system with the Blueberry Avocado Immunity Infusion. This smoothie combines the antioxidant power of blueberries with the creamy richness of avocado for a delicious and immune-boosting drink.

Total Prep Time: 7 minutes

Ingredients:
- 1/2 cup blueberries

- 1/2 avocado, peeled and pitted
- 1/2 cup spinach leaves
- 1 tablespoon honey
- 1 cup almond milk
- Ice cubes (optional)

Instructions:
1. Combine blueberries, avocado, spinach leaves, honey, and almond milk in a blender.
2. Blend until smooth and immune-boosting.
3. Pour into a glass and enjoy the Blueberry Avocado Immunity Infusion.

Information:
Calories: 180 | Protein: 4g | Fat: 8g | Carbohydrates: 25g | Fiber: 7g

Kale Pomegranate Powerhouse

Intro: Fuel your day with the nutrient-packed Kale Pomegranate Powerhouse. This green smoothie combines the powerhouse ingredients of kale and pomegranate for a vibrant and energizing drink.

Total Prep Time: 6 minutes

Ingredients:
- 1 cup kale, stems removed
- 1/2 cup pomegranate seeds
- 1/2 banana
- 1 tablespoon flaxseeds
- 1 cup coconut water
- Ice cubes (optional)

Instructions:
1. Combine kale, pomegranate seeds, banana, flaxseeds, and coconut water in a blender.
2. Blend until smooth and nutrient-packed.
3. Pour into a glass and enjoy the Kale Pomegranate Powerhouse.

Nutritional Information:
Calories: 150 | Protein: 3g | Fat: 3g | Carbohydrates: 30g | Fiber: 8g

Watercress Cucumber Hydration Shake

Intro: Stay hydrated with the Watercress Cucumber Hydration Shake. This light and refreshing smoothie combine the hydrating properties of cucumber with the nutrient density of watercress for a rejuvenating drink.

Total Prep Time: 5 minutes

Ingredients:
- 1/2 cucumber, peeled and sliced
- 1 cup watercress
- 1/2 apple, cored and chopped
- 1 tablespoon lemon juice
- 1 cup water
- Ice cubes (optional)

Instructions:
1. Combine cucumber, watercress, apple, lemon juice, and water in a blender.

2. Blend until smooth and hydrating.
3. Pour into a glass, garnish with a watercress sprig, and enjoy the Watercress Cucumber Hydration Shake.

Nutritional Information:
Calories: 80 | Protein: 2g | Fat: 0.5g | Carbohydrates: 20g | Fiber: 4g

Mixed Berry Chia Detox

Intro: Cleanse and rejuvenate with the Mixed Berry Chia Detox. This antioxidant-rich smoothie combines a medley of berries with the detoxifying benefits of chia seeds for a refreshing and revitalizing drink.

Total Prep Time: 8 minutes

Ingredients:
- 1/2 cup mixed berries (blueberries, strawberries, raspberries)
- 1 tablespoon chia seeds
- 1/2 cucumber, peeled and sliced
- 1 tablespoon mint leaves
- 1 cup coconut water
- Ice cubes (optional)

Instructions:
1. Combine mixed berries, chia seeds, cucumber, mint leaves, and coconut water in a blender.
2. Blend until smooth and detoxifying.
3. Pour into a glass and enjoy the Mixed Berry Chia Detox.

Calories: 120 | Protein: 3g | Fat: 3g |
Carbohydrates: 25g | Fiber: 8g

Apple Cinnamon Slimming Shake

Intro: Embrace the cozy flavors of fall with the Apple Cinnamon Slimming Shake. This smoothie is not only delicious but also supports your weight loss goals with the perfect blend of sweetness and spice.

Total Prep Time: 6 minutes

Ingredients:
- 1 apple, cored and sliced
- 1/2 teaspoon cinnamon
- 1/2 banana
- 1 cup almond milk
- 1 tablespoon chia seeds
- Ice cubes (optional)

Instructions:
1. Combine apple slices, cinnamon, banana, almond milk, and chia seeds in a blender.
2. Blend until smooth and slimming.
3. Pour into a glass, sprinkle a dash of cinnamon on top, and enjoy the Apple Cinnamon Slimming Shake.

Nutritional Information:
Calories: 180 | Protein: 3g | Fat: 5g |
Carbohydrates: 30g | Fiber: 8g

Vanilla Almond Joyful Blend

Intro*:* Indulge in the blissful combination of vanilla and almond with the Vanilla Almond Joyful Blend. This smoothie is a guilt-free treat that satisfies your sweet cravings while providing a dose of protein.

Total Prep Time*:* 5 minutes

Ingredients*:*
- 1/2 cup almonds, soaked
- 1/2 teaspoon vanilla extract
- 1 banana
- 1 cup almond milk
- 1 tablespoon shredded coconut
- Ice cubes (optional)

Instructions*:*
1. Combine soaked almonds, vanilla extract, banana, almond milk, and shredded coconut in a blender.
2. Blend until smooth and joyful.
3. Pour into a glass, sprinkle a bit of shredded coconut on top, and enjoy the Vanilla Almond Joyful Blend.

Nutritional Information*:*
Calories: 250 | Protein: 8g | Fat: 15g | Carbohydrates: 28g | Fiber: 7g

Spinach Pineapple Green Goddess

Intro*:* Channel the power of greens with the Spinach Pineapple Green Goddess smoothie. Packed with vitamins and minerals, this green elixir will make you feel vibrant and refreshed.

Total Prep Time*:* 7 minutes

Ingredients*:*
- 1 cup spinach leaves
- 1/2 cup pineapple chunks
- 1/2 banana
- 1 tablespoon ginger, grated
- 1 cup coconut water
- Ice cubes (optional)

Instructions*:*
1. Combine spinach leaves, pineapple chunks, banana, grated ginger, and coconut water in a blender.
2. Blend until smooth and goddess-worthy.
3. Pour into a glass, garnish with a pineapple slice, and enjoy the Spinach Pineapple Green Goddess.

Nutritional Information*:*
Calories: 140 | Protein: 2g | Fat: 1g | Carbohydrates: 35g | Fiber: 4g

Berry Beet Bliss

Intro: Experience the vibrant hues of the Berry Beet Bliss smoothie. This antioxidant-rich blend combines the sweetness of berries with the earthy goodness of beets for a blissful and nutritious drink.

Total Prep Time: 8 minutes

Ingredients:
- 1/2 cup mixed berries (blueberries, strawberries, raspberries)
- 1/2 cup beets, peeled and diced
- 1/2 cup Greek yogurt
- 1 tablespoon honey
- 1 cup water
- Ice cubes (optional)

Instructions:
1. Combine mixed berries, beets, Greek yogurt, honey, and water in a blender.
2. Blend until smooth and blissful.
3. Pour into a glass, garnish with a few berries, and enjoy the Berry Beet Bliss.

Nutritional Information:
Calories: 160 | Protein: 5g | Fat: 2g | Carbohydrates: 30g | Fiber: 7g

Mango Ginger Wellness Wonder

Intro: Boost your wellness with the Mango Ginger Wellness Wonder. This tropical smoothie combines the tropical sweetness of mango with the immune-boosting properties of ginger for a refreshing and revitalizing drink.

Total Prep Time*:* 6 minutes

Ingredients*:*
- 1 cup mango chunks
- 1/2 teaspoon ginger, grated
- 1/2 banana
- 1 tablespoon chia seeds
- 1 cup coconut water
- Ice cubes (optional)

Instructions*:*
1. Combine mango chunks, grated ginger, banana, chia seeds, and coconut water in a blender.
2. Blend until smooth and wellness-boosting.
3. Pour into a glass, garnish with a mango slice, and enjoy the Mango Ginger Wellness Wonder.

Nutritional Information*:*
Calories: 150 | Protein: 3g | Fat: 3g | Carbohydrates: 30g | Fiber: 7g

Cucumber Kiwi Cooling Cleanse

Intro*:* Cool down and cleanse with the Cucumber Kiwi Cooling Cleanse. This hydrating smoothie combines the crispness of cucumber with the tartness of kiwi for a refreshing and detoxifying experience.

Total Prep Time: 5 minutes

Ingredients:
- 1/2 cucumber, peeled and sliced
- 2 kiwis, peeled and sliced
- 1/2 lime, juiced
- 1 tablespoon mint leaves
- 1 cup water
- Ice cubes (optional)

Instructions:
1. Combine cucumber, kiwis, lime juice, mint leaves, and water in a blender.
2. Blend until smooth and cooling.
3. Pour into a glass, garnish with a kiwi slice, and enjoy the Cucumber Kiwi Cooling Cleanse.

Nutritional Information:
Calories: 80 | Protein: 2g | Fat: 0.5g | Carbohydrates: 20g | Fiber: 5g

Chocolate Peanut Butter Protein Bliss

Intro: Indulge in the decadent combination of chocolate and peanut butter with the Chocolate Peanut Butter Protein Bliss smoothie. This protein-packed treat is perfect for satisfying your cravings and fueling your day.

Total Prep Time: 6 minutes

Ingredients*:*
- 1 tablespoon cacao powder
- 2 tablespoons peanut butter
- 1 scoop chocolate protein powder
- 1 banana
- 1 cup almond milk
- Ice cubes (optional)

Instructions*:*
1. Combine cacao powder, peanut butter, chocolate protein powder, banana, and almond milk in a blender.
2. Blend until smooth and blissfully chocolatey.
3. Pour into a glass, drizzle with a bit of peanut butter, and enjoy the Chocolate Peanut Butter Protein Bliss.

Nutritional Information*:*
Calories: 270 | Protein: 20g | Fat: 12g | Carbohydrates: 30g | Fiber: 7g

Matcha Green Tea Fat Burner

Intro*:* Boost your metabolism with the Matcha Green Tea Fat Burner. This smoothie combines the antioxidant-rich properties of matcha with other fat-burning ingredients for a delicious and energizing drink.

Total Prep Time*:* 7 minutes

Ingredients*:*
- 1 teaspoon matcha powder
- 1/2 cup pineapple chunks
- 1/2 banana
- 1 tablespoon chia seeds
- 1 cup green tea, brewed and cooled
- Ice cubes (optional)

Instructions*:*
1. Combine matcha powder, pineapple chunks, banana, chia seeds, and green tea in a blender.
2. Blend until smooth and fat-burning.
3. Pour into a glass, garnish with a pineapple slice, and enjoy the Matcha Green Tea Fat Burner.

Nutritional Information*:*
Calories: 120 | Protein: 3g | Fat: 2g | Carbohydrates: 25g | Fiber: 6g

Pineapple Mango Mint Slim Down

Intro*:* Support your slimming goals with the Pineapple Mango Mint Slim Down. This tropical smoothie combines the sweetness of pineapple and mango with the refreshing essence of mint for a delightful and slimming experience.

Total Prep Time*:* 6 minutes

Ingredients*:*
- 1/2 cup pineapple chunks
- 1/2 cup mango chunks
- 1/4 cup fresh mint leaves

- 1/2 lime, juiced
- 1 cup coconut water
- Ice cubes (optional)

Instructions:
1. Combine pineapple chunks, mango chunks, fresh mint leaves, lime juice, and coconut water in a blender.
2. Blend until smooth and slimming.
3. Pour into a glass, garnish with a mint sprig, and enjoy the Pineapple Mango Mint Slim Down.

Nutritional Information:
Calories: 140 | Protein: 1g | Fat: 0.5g | Carbohydrates: 35g | Fiber: 4g

Raspberry Coconut Refresher

Intro: Refresh your senses with the Raspberry Coconut Refresher. This smoothie combines the tartness of raspberries with the tropical creaminess of coconut for a revitalizing and hydrating experience.

Total Prep Time: 5 minutes

Ingredients:
- 1/2 cup raspberries
- 1/2 cup coconut milk
- 1/2 banana
- 1 tablespoon honey
- 1 cup ice cubes

***Instructions*:**
1. Combine raspberries, coconut milk, banana, honey, and ice cubes in a blender.
2. Blend until smooth and refreshing.
3. Pour into a glass, garnish with a few raspberries, and enjoy the Raspberry Coconut Refresher.

***Nutritional Information*:**
Calories: 150 | Protein: 2g | Fat: 7g | Carbohydrates: 25g | Fiber: 5g

Peach Basil Beauty Boost

***Intro*:** Enhance your natural beauty with the Peach Basil Beauty Boost. This delightful smoothie combines the sweet essence of peaches with the aromatic touch of basil, providing a beauty-enhancing treat.

***Total Prep Time*:** 6 minutes

***Ingredients*:**
- 1 cup peaches, sliced
- 1/2 cup basil leaves
- 1/2 cup Greek yogurt
- 1 tablespoon honey
- 1 cup water
- Ice cubes (optional)

***Instructions*:**
1. Combine peaches, basil leaves, Greek yogurt, honey, and water in a blender.
2. Blend until smooth and beauty-boosting.

3. Pour into a glass, garnish with a basil leaf, and enjoy the Peach Basil Beauty Boost.

Nutritional Information:
Calories: 140 | Protein: 5g | Fat: 2g | Carbohydrates: 25g | Fiber: 4g

Blueberry Avocado Alkalizer

Intro: Balance your body's pH levels with the Blueberry Avocado Alkalizer. This smoothie combines the antioxidant-rich blueberries with the creamy goodness of avocado, creating a delicious and alkalizing drink.

Total Prep Time: 7 minutes

Ingredients:
- 1/2 cup blueberries
- 1/2 avocado, peeled and pitted
- 1/2 cup kale, stems removed
- 1 tablespoon lemon juice
- 1 cup coconut water
- Ice cubes (optional)

Instructions:
1. Combine blueberries, avocado, kale, lemon juice, and coconut water in a blender.
2. Blend until smooth and alkalizing.
3. Pour into a glass and enjoy the Blueberry Avocado Alkalizer.

Nutritional Information:
Calories: 160 | Protein: 3g | Fat: 8g | Carbohydrates: 25g | Fiber: 7g

Turmeric Citrus Detox Elixir

Intro*:* Detoxify your body with the Turmeric Citrus Detox Elixir. This vibrant smoothie combines the anti-inflammatory properties of turmeric with the refreshing essence of citrus fruits for a detoxifying and immune-boosting drink.

Total Prep Time*:* 8 minutes

Ingredients*:*
- 1/2 teaspoon turmeric powder
- 1/2 orange, peeled and segmented
- 1/2 grapefruit, peeled and segmented
- 1 tablespoon chia seeds
- 1 cup coconut water
- Ice cubes (optional)

Instructions*:*
1. Combine turmeric powder, orange segments, grapefruit segments, chia seeds, and coconut water in a blender.
2. Blend until smooth and detoxifying.
3. Pour into a glass, garnish with an orange slice, and enjoy the Turmeric Citrus Detox Elixir.

Nutritional Information:
Calories: 120 | Protein: 3g | Fat: 2g | Carbohydrates: 25g | Fiber: 6g

Strawberry Kiwi Fat Flush

Intro*:* Give your body a boost with the Strawberry Kiwi Fat Flush. This smoothie combines the sweetness of strawberries with the tartness of kiwi, creating a refreshing and fat-flushing drink to support your wellness goals.

Total Prep Time*:* 6 minutes

Ingredients*:*
- 1 cup strawberries, hulled
- 2 kiwis, peeled and sliced
- 1/2 cucumber, peeled and sliced
- 1 tablespoon mint leaves
- 1 cup water
- Ice cubes (optional)

Instructions*:*
1. Combine strawberries, kiwis, cucumber, mint leaves, and water in a blender.
2. Blend until smooth and fat-flushing.
3. Pour into a glass, garnish with a strawberry slice, and enjoy the Strawberry Kiwi Fat Flush.

Nutritional Information*:*
Calories: 90 | Protein: 2g | Fat: 0.5g | Carbohydrates: 22g | Fiber: 6g

Blackberry Spinach Antioxidant Shake

Intro: Boost your antioxidant intake with the Blackberry Spinach Antioxidant Shake. This green smoothie combines the richness of blackberries with the nutrient density of spinach for a delicious and antioxidant-packed drink.

Total Prep Time: 7 minutes

Ingredients:
- 1/2 cup blackberries
- 1 cup spinach leaves
- 1/2 banana
- 1 tablespoon almond butter
- 1 cup almond milk
- Ice cubes (optional)

Instructions:
1. Combine blackberries, spinach leaves, banana, almond butter, and almond milk in a blender.
2. Blend until smooth and antioxidant-rich.
3. Pour into a glass and enjoy the Blackberry Spinach Antioxidant Shake.

Nutritional Information:
Calories: 160 | Protein: 5g | Fat: 8g | Carbohydrates: 25g | Fiber: 7g

Ginger Pear Metabolism Booster

Intro: Fire up your metabolism with the Ginger Pear Metabolism Booster. This smoothie combines the zesty kick of ginger with the sweetness of pear for a metabolism-boosting and energizing drink.

Total Prep Time: 6 minutes

Ingredients:
- 1 pear, cored and sliced
- 1/2 teaspoon ginger, grated
- 1/2 banana
- 1 tablespoon honey
- 1 cup water
- Ice cubes (optional)

Instructions:
1. Combine pear slices, grated ginger, banana, honey, and water in a blender.
2. Blend until smooth and metabolism-boosting.
3. Pour into a glass, garnish with a pear slice, and enjoy the Ginger Pear Metabolism Booster.

Nutritional Information:
Calories: 120 | Protein: 1g | Fat: 0.5g | Carbohydrates: 30g | Fiber: 6g

Watermelon Mint Hydration Elixir

Intro: Stay hydrated with the Watermelon Mint Hydration Elixir. This light and refreshing smoothie combine the hydrating properties of watermelon with the invigorating essence of mint for a revitalizing and hydrating drink.

Total Prep Time: 5 minutes

Ingredients:
- 1 cup watermelon, cubed
- 1/4 cup fresh mint leaves
- 1/2 lime, juiced
- 1 cup coconut water
- Ice cubes (optional)

Instructions:
1. Combine watermelon, fresh mint leaves, lime juice, and coconut water in a blender.
2. Blend until smooth and hydrating.
3. Pour into a glass, garnish with a watermelon wedge, and enjoy the Watermelon Mint Hydration Elixir.

Nutritional Information:
Calories: 70 | Protein: 1g | Fat: 0.5g | Carbohydrates: 18g | Fiber: 3g

Banana Berry Protein Powerhouse

Intro: Fuel your day with the Banana Berry Protein Powerhouse. This protein-packed smoothie combines the sweetness of bananas with a medley of berries for a satisfying and energizing drink.

Total Prep Time: 6 minutes

Ingredients:
- 1 banana
- 1/2 cup mixed berries (blueberries, strawberries, raspberries)
- 1 scoop vanilla protein powder
- 1 tablespoon almond butter
- 1 cup almond milk
- Ice cubes (optional)

Instructions:
1. Combine banana, mixed berries, vanilla protein powder, almond butter, and almond milk in a blender.
2. Blend until smooth and protein-packed.
3. Pour into a glass, drizzle with a bit of almond butter, and enjoy the Banana Berry Protein Powerhouse.

Nutritional Information:
Calories: 260 | Protein: 18g | Fat: 10g | Carbohydrates: 30g | Fiber: 7g

Kiwi Orange Vitamin C Infusion

Intro*:* Boost your immune system with the Kiwi Orange Vitamin C Infusion. This citrusy smoothie combines the vitamin C-rich goodness of kiwi and oranges for an immune-boosting and refreshing drink.

Total Prep Time*:* 5 minutes

Ingredients*:*
- 2 kiwis, peeled and sliced
- 1 orange, peeled and segmented
- 1/2 lemon, juiced
- 1 tablespoon honey
- 1 cup water
- Ice cubes (optional)

Instructions*:*
1. Combine kiwis, orange segments, lemon juice, honey, and water in a blender.
2. Blend until smooth and vitamin C-infused.
3. Pour into a glass, garnish with a kiwi slice, and enjoy the Kiwi Orange Vitamin C Infusion.

Nutritional Information*:*
Calories: 90 | Protein: 1g | Fat: 0.5g | Carbohydrates: 22g | Fiber: 5g

Mixed Berry Oatmeal Smoothie

Intro: Start your day right with the Mixed Berry Oatmeal Smoothie. This wholesome blend combines the goodness of mixed berries with the heartiness of oats for a satisfying and nutritious breakfast in a glass.

Total Prep Time: 8 minutes

Ingredients:
- 1/2 cup mixed berries (blueberries, strawberries, raspberries)
- 1/4 cup oats
- 1/2 banana
- 1 tablespoon Greek yoghourt
- 1 cup almond milk
- Ice cubes (optional)

Instructions:
1. Combine mixed berries, oats, banana, Greek yoghourt, and almond milk in a blender.
2. Blend until smooth and oatmeal-infused.
3. Pour into a glass, sprinkle a few oats on top, and enjoy the Mixed Berry Oatmeal Smoothie.

Nutritional Information:
Calories: 180 | Protein: 5g | Fat: 3g | Carbohydrates: 35g | Fiber: 8g

www.ingramcontent.com/pod-product-compliance
Lightning Source LLC
Chambersburg PA
CBHW070735260726
48660CB00007B/2850